ARE YOU WHAT YOU EAT?

Why Your Intestines Are The Foundation of Good Health

Holly Fourchalk, PhD., DNM®, RHT, HT

CHOICES UNLIMITED

FOR

HEALTH AND WELLNESS

Dr. Holly Fourchalk, Ph.D., DNM®, RHT, HT

Tel: 604.764.5203
Fax: 604.465.7964

Website: www.choicesunlimited.ca
E-mail: holly@choicesunlimited.ca

Editing, Interior Design and Cover Design:
Wendy Dewar Hughes, Summer Bay Press

ISBN: 978-1-927626-30-6
Digital ISBN: 978-1-927626-31-3

This book includes neither an exhaustive nor exclusive list of alternative options for working with adrenal fatigue.

Rather, it provides an overview of theories, foods, herbs and modalities with which the patient or practitioner may work.

My company is called Choices Unlimited for Health and Wellness for a reason. There are lots of choices to choose from with regard to maximizing your health. We can only make good, effective choices when we have a working knowledge of what those choices may be.

If a given modality or protocol resonates for you, research it further. Explore your options within the profile. Your mind is a very powerful tool – make it work for you. Regardless of what you choose to do, make the placebo effect – or the power of the mind – be a part of your healing journey.

Here's to your journey into health.

DISCLAIMER

Every effort has been made by the author to ensure that the information in this book is as accurate as possible. However, it is by no means a complete or exhaustive examination of all information.

The author knows what worked for her and what has worked for others but no two people are the same and so the author cannot and does not render judgment or advice regarding a particular individual.

Further, because our bodies are unique any two individuals may experience different results from the same therapy.

The author believes in both prevention and the superiority of a natural non-invasive approach over drugs and surgery.

The information collected within comes from a variety of researchers and sources from around the world. This information has been accumulated in the Western healing arts over the past thirty years.

Research has shown that one of the top three leading causes of death in North America occurs because of the physician/pharmaceutical component of the scenario.

Perhaps the real leading cause of death and disability is a result of the lack of awareness of natural therapies. These therapies are well known to prevent and treat many common degenerative, inflammatory and oxidative diseases.

The author loves to research and loves to teach. This book is another attempt to increase awareness about health and the many options we have to bring the body back into a healthy balance.

Ever-increasing numbers of people are aware of healing foods and herbs, supplements and modalities but there are still far too many who are not. The fact that our physicians are part of this latter group makes healing even more challenging yet we are now seeing more and more laboratories around the world and more universities in and outside of the U.S. studying herbs, nutrition and various healing modalities with phenomenal success.

The unfortunate fact is, those who can profit from sickness and disease promote ignorance and the results are devastating.

It is not the intent of the author that anyone should choose to read this book and make decisions regarding their health or medical care based on ideas contained in this book.

It is the responsibility of the individual to find a health care practitioner to work with to achieve optimal health.

The author and publisher are not responsible for any adverse effects or consequences resulting from the use of any of the suggestions or information contained in the book but offer this material as information that the public has a right to hear and utilize at its own discretion.

To my Parents

For all their support and encouragement
My Dad for his ever-listening ear
My mother for her open mind

CONTENTS

PART ONE

ONE

Your gut is not really part of your body....

"All disease begins in the gut."

Hippocrates

Have you ever thought of this? Your whole intestinal tract from your mouth down to your anus is outside of your body. It is a long tube, with a number of different components that runs through your body but inside of the tube, you are actually outside of the body.

This tube is called the GIT or gastro-intestinal tract. This book is designed to help you understand that tube, the GIT, which runs through you, and how dysfunctions in your GIT can affect every other system in the body.

For easy reference, the book is divided into three parts:

Part I will explore the digestive tract – what is does and of what it is composed.

Part II will explore dysfunctions in the digestive tract and how those impact different parts of the body.

Part III will explore what we need to do to maintain a good healthy digestive tract or recover when the digestive tract is not functioning properly.

The book is organized so that you do not have to read Chapter One to understand Chapter Five; rather, go to the parts of the book that interest you the most and then go back to the parts that will give you further understanding.

Let's look at this tube we each have a little more closely.

It starts with your mouth. Your mouth is not simply something you eat and taste with. Your mouth, or the buccal cavity, is the first complex, dynamic component of the GIT.

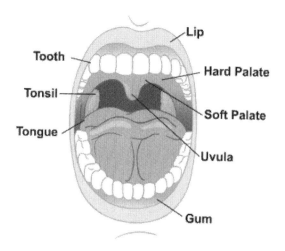

The mouth contains, not only teeth, a tongue and saliva (between 1 – 1.5 litres/day) to chew your food with but it also contains:

Exocrine glands:

- 3 pairs (parotid, submandibular and sublingual) that secrete saliva
- Saliva contains digestive enzymes:
- amylase which breaks down carbohydrates
- lipase which breaks down fats
- Mucus: helps to soften foods

Blood vessels:

The mouth and its structures require a fair amount of blood flow and are consequently highly vascularized, or loaded with blood vessels. These blood vessels, the arteries, bring nutrients and the veins take away toxins to and from the tongue, lips, teeth and gums, palate, and glands.

Lymph system:

Usually, the lymphatic system parallels the blood system. There is a lymphatic system that runs through your mouth, at the upper lip and teeth, the outside or lateral parts of the front of the tongue, plus the submandibular lymph nodes and the submental lymph nodes.

Nerves:

There are twelve cranial nerves in the brain. Many of these serve the mouth in some way, both for sensory (receive information) and motor information. The most important ones are:

- Trigeminal: 5th
- Facial: 8th
- Glossopharyngeal: 9th
- Hypoglossal: 12th

Uvula:

The uvula is a projection that hangs down from the roof of the mouth and contains both glands and muscular fibres, and is also involved in the production of speech.

Bacteria:

Like the rest of the GIT, the mouth has bacteria that are referred to as the microflora. There are five categories of oral bacteria:

- Streptococci
- Lactobacilli
- Staphylococci
- Corynebacteria,
- Bacteroide

Each category has numerous subcategories. Most of the bacteria that evolve in the mouth (newborns do not have bacteria in their mouths) develop rapidly during the first few weeks of newborn life. As we move into puberty we gain even new ones. These good bacteria require a good pH balance to survive. If the pH of the mouth becomes too acidic, bacteria that we don't want start to thrive.

Unfortunately, if we are not careful, we can also support other bacteria that cause problems in our mouth, for instance:

- Treponema denticola: Develop with various dental diseases.
- Fusospirochetes: Thrive when there is bleeding and can cause infections.
- Veillonella: Thrives in acidic environments.
- Porphyromonas gingivalis: Associated with chronic adult periodontitis (inflammation of the tissues that support the teeth).
- Aggregatibacter actinomycetemcomitans: Cause both inflammation and bone deterioration.
- Lactobacillu: Associated with dental caries or dental cavities – usually found in the gut flora.

From your mouth we now travel down the throat. We know that when we chew food, we have to swallow and it goes down the throat. The throat is another complex pieces of equipment.

Both our air and our food go down that tunnel. The throat's primary features consist of the following.

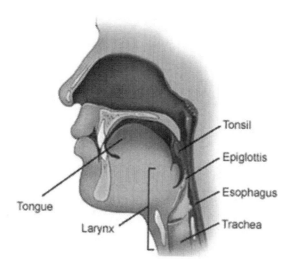

Tonsil

Epiglottis

Esophagus

Trachea

Tongue

Larynx

Tonsils:

Part of the lymphatic/immune system, which includes adenoid tonsils, tubal tonsils, palatine tonsils and lingual tonsils, and lie behind and to the sides of uvula.

Hyoid bone:

A bone shaped like a horseshoe that lies at the base of mouth forming the lower jaw.

Pharynx:

Part of both the respiratory and the digestive system and important in vocalization.

Larynx:

Situated underneath the pharynx where the throat splits into the trachea and esophagus. The vocal cords, or the voice box, are located in the larynx and involved in both pitch and volume of the voice. It is part of the respiratory system and protects the trachea from food.

Trachea:

Connects the pharynx to the larynx.

Thyroid:

A butterfly shaped organ that lies both against and around the larynx and trachea. Its primary functions are to produce the hormones T3, T4, and calcitonin.

Parathyroid:

Usually four small endocrine/hormonal glands that secrete parathyroid hormone in response to the amount of calcium that they monitor in the blood.

Epiglottis:

Is a flap made of elastic cartilage and attached to the entrance of the larynx. We have taste buds even here. The epiglottis guards the entrance to the glottis and is one of nine cartilage-like structures that make up the voice box.

Esophagus:

Is a muscular tube. Food passes through the pharynx and down the esophagus, through the lower esophageal sphincter/valves into the stomach.

Blood:

The carotid arteries bring blood, oxygen and nutrients to the neck, head, mouth and brain. The jugular veins bring the blood vessels, depleted of oxygen and full of toxins, down from the head and neck back to the heart.

Nerves:

The three predominant nerves that go through the neck are:

- Phrenic: originates in the neck
- Glossopharyngeal: 9th
- Vagus: 10th
- Accessory: 11th
- Hypoglossal: 12th

Lymph:

Like the mouth, the neck is lined with lymph nodes. The lymph nodes are filled with a fluid that contains lymphocytes (white blood cells) that make anti-bodies in response to pathogens in the system. If there is an increase in the number of immune cells fighting an infection, the node may become swollen. The nodes in the neck are:

- Under the jaw
- Either side of the neck
- Behind the ears

One can easily see that the throat is not a simple channel for food to go down but rather another complex component of the GIT.

Stomach

How come everyone pats his or her belly when speaking of a full stomach? The stomach does not reside in the belly region. It resides under the heart.

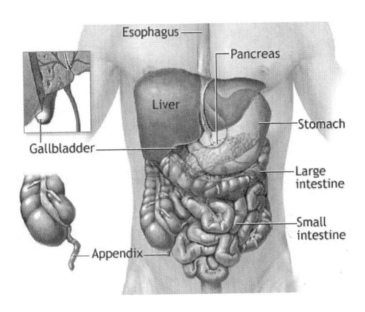

But let's look at the stomach itself. This is the most acidic part of the body with a pH that can go as low as 1.2. The stomach is basically a muscular but hollow sausage tube. This is where the second stage of digestion begins. The hydrochloric acid in the stomach breaks down food, and in particular proteins, into a pulp called chyme and then sends the chyme into the small intestine.

The stomach has 4 primary different regions:

Cardia:

This is where the esophageal sphincter releases food into the stomach.

Fundus:

This is the upper curve of the stomach and is used to store some foods, while the stomach is digesting other foods. For instance, fruit may get pushed up here, while the body of the stomach digests proteins.

Body:

This is where the majority of the digestive process occurs.

Pyloric:

This is the lower section that helps to alkalize the

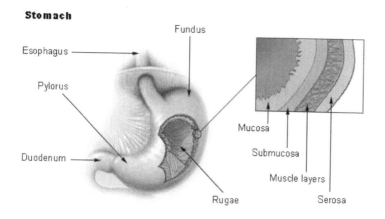

Stomach

Esophagus

Pylorus

Duodenum

Fundus

Rugae

Mucosa

Submucosa

Muscle layers

Serosa

chyme before it goes into the small intestine.

Layers of the stomach:

There are four major layers to the stomach wall as can be seen above. These layers both produce and protect.

The first layer of the stomach walls is called the mucosa and as its name suggests, produces mucus. This layer also contains a type of muscle called a smooth muscle.

The submucosa layer has a fibrous connective tissue, which means it contains cells, fibres, body fluids and what is called extracellular matrices. This layer also houses the nerves for the stomach in what is called the Meissner's plexus.

The third layer is called the muscularis externa – which contains three layers of smooth muscle (the rest contains only two layers of smooth muscles).

The fourth layer is called the serosa and is made up of connective tissues that connect with the peritoneum – the muscles that go around the entire abdominal cavity.

Blood:

Like all parts of the body and GIT, the stomach requires an ongoing blood supply. The stomach has a few different arterial supplies:

- Gastric artery
- Celiac trunk

- Gastroduodenal artery

Glands:

There are three types of glands in the stomach and they are found in the following.

- *Cardia:* Cardiac glands secrete mucus.
- *Fundus:* Fundic glands secrete mucus, gastric acid, IF (intrinsic factor), pepsinogen (helps to break down proteins into peptides), rennin (in newborns to curdle the milk) and hormones.
- *Pylorus*: Pyloric glands contain both mucus cells and G cells and secrete gastrin.

Fluids:

- *Gastric acid:* Made up of hydrochloric acid, it acidifies the stomach, pH = 1-2. Helps to protect the system against pathogens.
- *Hydrochloric acid*: A solution of hydrogen and chloride in water. Breaks down proteins.
- *Pepsin* : an enzyme released into the stomach to break down food proteins into peptides
- *Mucin* : helps to form the mucosal gel that protects the lining
- Intrinsic Factor (IF): necessary to absorb Vitamin B12

Nerves:

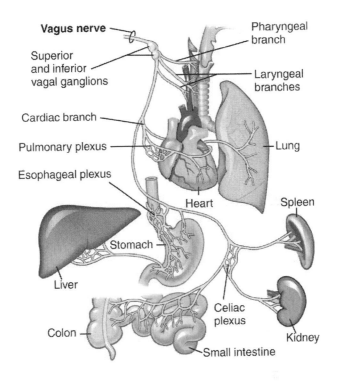

Small Intestine:

The small intestine follows the stomach and is where much of the digestive processes and absorption processes occur. The average length of the small intestine is thought to be about 22.5 feet long or 6.9 metres in adult males and 23.5 feet, or 7.16 metres, long in adult females. However, this length can range from about 15 – 32 feet long (4.6 – 9.75 metres). How long do you think yours is?

There are three major components to the small intestine:

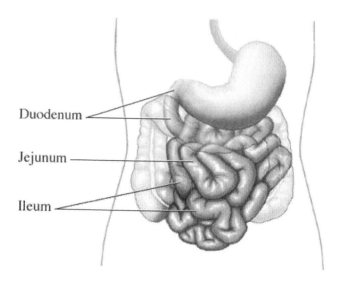

Duodenum
Jejunum
Ileum

Duodenum:

The first part that receives the chyme from the stomach; it is the shortest part and where most of the digestive processes occur. The cells secrete secretin and cholecystokinin, which provoke the liver and gallbladder to release bile and the pancreas to release bicarbonate and digestive enzymes (trypsin, lipase, amylase).

Jejunum:

The second part of the small intestine has a pH between 7 and 9. It contains both circular and longitudinal smooth muscles, which help to move the food along through a movement called peristalsis.

This area absorbs a wide variety of nutrients (sugars, amino acids, vitamins) that were digested in the duodenum, but not fat.

Ileum:

The last part of the small intestine has a pH between 7 and 8; it absorbs B12 and bile salts. Its cells secrete hormones (gastrin, secretin, cholescystokinin) and enzymes (protease and carbohydrase).

The small intestine has three major sources of contribution:

- *Chyme:* from the stomach
- *Bile:* from the gallbladder/liver
- *Hormones and Enzymes:* from the pancreas

Large Intestine:

This is the last part of the GIT and the home of the majority of microbiota in the body. There are approximately ten times more bacteria than cells in the body and the majority of them are located in the colon. The colon's primary function is to absorb water from the remaining food particles, not digested. It also absorbs vitamins like Vitamin K (created by bacteria), Vitamin B1, B2, B12. The large intestine is also responsible for the fermentation of carbohydrates. Fatty acids and uric acid also occur in the colon. It is also responsible for both moving and compacting the feces.

The pH of the large intestine runs between 5.5 and 7. On average, the large intestine is about 5 feet, or 1.5 metres, long. There are five major parts to the large intestine:

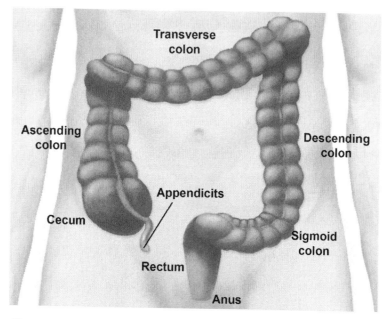

Cecum:

A small pouch that identifies the beginning of the large intestine, it produces enzymes that break down fats, and bacteria that break down plant cellulose. While most gut bacteria are anaerobes (they don't like oxygen), bacteria in the cecum are aerobic (they require oxygen).

Appendix:

A small pouch that is part of the lymphatic system, with a high amount of lymphoid cells (which fight infection), it is believed that the appendix holds extra bacteria as a back up for when it is needed.

Colon:

Composed of the ascending, transverse and descending components and the sigmoid colon, the colon receives fluid from the small intestine and extracts water and salt turning the fluid into a solid stool. Sodium and some fat-soluble vitamins are absorbed. Bacteria in the colon (over 700 bacteria) digest fibre as food and create acetate, propionate and butyrate, which are then used by the cells in the lining for food.

Rectum:

When the feces reach the rectum, the stretch receptors trigger the desire to defecate. If you don't defecate at this point, the material returns to the prior segment. The longer the delay occurs, the more likely you will build up hard

ened feces and become constipated.

Anal canal: The last part of the large intestine, it is only a couple of inches long.

The large intestine produces two fluids:

- Potassium
- Chloride

Bacteria:

There are over 700 identified bacteria in the large intestine. The entire digestive tract is coated with a bacterial layer that provides natural protection to invading organisms, undigested food, toxins and parasites. There is between 3 and 4.5 pounds of bacteria in the gut or, about one billion bacteria per gram of large bowel content.

These bacteria are very important to our health, to the point that some have suggested that these bacteria could be considered as a separate metabolic organ in the body. Some of the functions they are required for are:

- Digestion of food through fermentation.
- Neutralizing harmful by-products of digestion.
- Help with the absorption of nutrients.
- Producing required vitamins we don't get in our diet, i.e. Vitamin K, as well as, producing Vitamins B1, B2, B3, B5, B6 and B12.
- Contribute to the immune system:
  - Form the first line of defense against "bad bacteria" by :
    - competing for food
    - effecting the oxygen levels
    - adjusting the pH levels.
  - About 60% of the immune receptor cells are in the large intestine.

- o About 15% of these immune receptor cells are in the lower part of the small intestine.
- o Together, about 75% of the immune receptor cells are in the gut.
- o They trigger the production of a wide range of immune cells:
  - Neutrophils
  - Macrophages
  - Immune-globulins
  - Interferons
  - Interleukin-1
  - TNF – tumor necrosis factor

So let's put all this together and we have:

Organs of the Digestive System

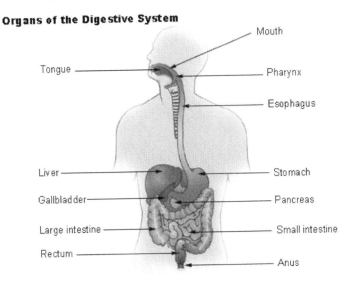

While this is just a general overview of the gastrointestinal structure and function, it provides a basic understanding of the complexity of the system. Now we will look at what happens when any component goes wrong.

TWO

Why your gut needs to function properly.

Now we know that we each have this tube that goes through our bodies. This tube has a number of different components. Each component functions in different ways to achieve different results. But why do we need this tube in us?

We don't just eat food because it tastes good, is a social activity, or because our gut tells us we are hungry. Let's look at some of the requirements we need food for:

- Blood – every cell in your body gets nutrients from blood – about 5 liters in an adult body – created from bone.
  - About 3 liters is plasma.
  - Between 4,500,000 (female) and 5,200,000 (male) red blood cells per microliter of blood and account for about 45% of the blood.
  - Between 4-10,000 white blood cells per microliter of blood.
  - About 600 red blood cells for every white blood cell.

- We make about 2-3 billion red blood cells per minute.
- We make 6 main categories of white blood cells: neutrophils, eosinophils, basophils, bands, monocytes, lymphocytes.

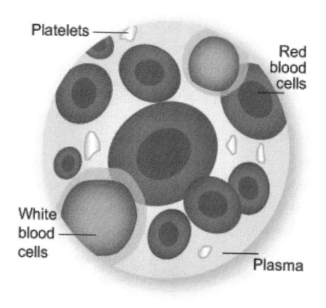

- Constantly make fuel in every cell of the body (in order to break anything down; build anything up; we need enzymes and enzymes need fuel/ATP.
- Repeatedly create over 10,000 different enzymes.
- Constantly replicate cells and eliminate the old ones.

- Create all the organelles within a cell
- Create a cell membrane with receptors and transporters.
- Create the tools for the cells to function.
- Constantly produce and repair over 29 different types of collagen.
  - The basis of bones, cartilage, tendons, ligaments, hair, nails, skin, membranes, etc.
- Synthesize over 100 different types of neurotransmitters.
  - Neurotransmitters are made both in the gut and in the brain.
  - The gut sometimes makes more neurotransmitters than the brain does, i.e. 98% of serotonin is made in the gut.
- Create over 50 different types of hormones.
  - Hormones may communicate from cell to cell, tissue to tissue, or organ to organ.
  - Hormones are involved in the cardio, reproductive, digestive, immune system, and skeletal, neurological, kidney, thyroid, adrenal and pancreatic systems.
- Create transport mechanisms to move nutrients and compounds from the gut to the blood and from the blood to the cells and then movement within the cells.

- Create anti-oxidants, i.e. glutathione, superoxide dismutase, catalase.
- Create inflammatory regulators and anti-inflammatories, i.e. prostaglandins, NF-kB.
- Create fatty acids, for instance, the acetyl coenzyme A that is required to make our fuel/ATP.
- Create lipids and cholesterol.
- Turn over bone.
- Breakdown cells, compounds, neurotransmitters, etc.
- Eliminate: old cells, by products and toxins (POPs, PCBs, heavy metals, etc.).
- ...and much more.

Obviously we need nutrients for the body to function. We need a good functioning gut to metabolize, synthesize and absorb all the nutrients the body requires to make all these components on an ongoing basis.

We need good nutrient for the gastrointestinal tract and the body to function well. Poor nutrients, like microwaved, pasteurized or processed nutrients simply deplete the body even further.

Now, can you imagine what might happen if:

- The gut is inflamed?
- The gut lining has holes in it?

- The pH level is too low for the enzymes to work?
- There is insufficient fibre (prebiotic) to feed the bacteria/probiotic?
- Toxicity is plugging up the cells, receptors and transporters?
- The immune system is broken down and pathogens are swarming and eating the very nutrient we need to survive?
- Pathogens are moving from the gut system into the blood and organs?
- Nutrients are not getting broken down?
- Toxicity is seeping through?

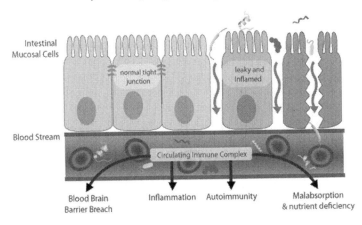

And the list can go on and on. Naturally, an unlimited number of functions can go wrong affecting every system in the body.

- Neurological (brain, spinal cord, peripheral nervous system)

- Respiratory (nasal, pharynx, larynx, bronchi, lungs, diaphragm)
- Immunological
- Cardio (heart, blood)
- Hepatic (liver)
- Lymphatic (lymph, lymph nodes, lymph glands)
- Endocrine (hormones, glands (hypothalamus, pituitary, pineal, thyroid, parathyroid, adrenals)
- Skeletal (bones, muscles, cartilage, ligaments, tendons)
- Integumentary (skin, hair, nails)
- Reproductive (sex organs: ovaries, fallopian tubes, uterus, vagina, breasts; testes, vas deferens, prostate)
- Urinary (Kidneys, ureters, bladder)

If we don't have a good gut and good nutrients can anything go wrong? You bet!

Now, I know you are going to say, "Yeah but, I know so and so, and they have had a horrible diet, and they drink and they are healthy!"

My answer is, they may not have symptoms but they are probably not healthy. You see, the body has a huge number of compensating systems and as long as it can keep compensating we don't notice symptoms in our western culture. When the body can't compensate any longer, that's when we end up at the doctor's office. He or she gives us medication to stop the symptoms but rarely does that actually solve the underlying issues causing the problems.

The underlying problem keeps getting worse; the medication depletes the body of nutrients and we end up on a cocktail of drugs.

Now, we may be one of the lucky ones who has a huge number of compensatory systems and the body can adapt and adapt and we die before the body stops compensating. But the vast majority of people are going to have problems long before that happens.

Also note, I said "western culture". That is because in many other cultures, they are taught to be aware when the body starts to compensate and to have the issues addressed right away so that they don't end up with the problems we have.

In many alternative/traditional medicines, there are six stages of disease. People learn to recognize disease or disharmony in the body at stage 1 and 2 and see the physician right away. Then they take the appropriate herbs and foods to correct the problem before it gets out of hand.

In our western culture, we don't even go to the doctor until we are in Stage 5, or sometimes even going into Stage 6. The conventional doctor does not look at how the body is functioning and what the body requires to intake or eliminate to function properly. Rather the conventional doctor looks at the symptoms and prescribes a man-made synthetic compound to cover up the symptoms. Bizarre!

The Six Stages of Disease

Accumulation	A system overloads	Usually issues in the gut: stomach, small or large intestine
Aggravation/ provocation	One system spills into another system	Spill into another part of the gut
Dissemination /migration	Vague low grade non-specific symptoms	Starts to spread outside of the gut
Localization/ deposition	Toxin accumulation	Overflow of toxins lead to malfunction and structural damage
Manifestation	Now identifiable symptoms	Symptoms begin to appear as disease
Chronicity/ Disruption	Natural repair mechanisms not able to reverse the issue	Disease becomes chronic

In addition, when the body is doing what it was designed to do we are taught to stop it. For instance, if we get a pathogen that has taken up residence, the immune system will burn it out with a fever, or flush it out with mucus, or wash it out with diarrhea. This is a good thing. But we have been taught that if the body talks and tries to do what it was designed to do to protect us we have to find an MD and stop the body from functioning in healthy way. The antibiotics that are then typically prescribed kill all the good bacteria that are in our gut – that we need – and our own immune system becomes compromised!

PART II

THREE

Your gut flora and microbes

We used to call the bacteria in the GIT, the gut flora but now we call the gut flora microbiota. As mentioned in Chapter One, there are over one thousand species of bacteria in the gut, although the current consensus is that the majority of the gut bacteria come from thirty to forty species.

There are actually tens of trillions of microorganisms in our intestines. It is estimated that they contain more than 3 million genes, which is about 150 times more than our total count of genes!

Further, this load of bacteria we carry around with us, can weigh as much as 2 kg!

Now, for the really interesting part: About one third of our gut flora or microbiota is the same as what most people have. The remaining two thirds tends to be unique to each of us. Factors that impact your particular microbiota include diet and supplements.

You already knew that your fingerprint is unique to you but did you know that your microbiota is unique to you, too?

All of these unique little characters contribute to the same functions:

- Help the body digest food that we have not been able to digest.
- Changes food into nutrients that we require.
- Contribute to intestinal development and function.
- Help regulate the epithelial lining of the intestines.
- Help our bodies keep control over micro-organisms that we don't want.
- Help to maintain the mucosal membrane that lines the intestinal walls.
- Help to move the stool through the large intestine.
- Play a big part in our immune system and immune modulation/regulation.
- Also play a part in drug metabolism.
- Breaks down dietary toxins
- Break down carcinogens.
- Assist in absorption of electrolytes.
- Assist in absorption of trace minerals.
- Their feeding on the fibre then allows the fibres to absorb toxins, recycle bile acids and cholesterol and take part in electrolyte and water metabolism.[1,2]

In consideration of how big a role this microbiota plays in maintaining our health and well being, scientists are now considering the gut microbiota as its own organ. As we are not born with the microbiota but acquire it as babies, it is being referred to as the "acquired" organ.

This microbiota starts to develop during birth. The microbiota of the infant was historically thought to be similar to the mother's because most bacterial species are acquired during birthing. However, we now know that a child's stool samples of bacteria (your stool should be about 60% bacteria) is not any more similar to their own parent than to any other adult.[3]

The infant's bacterial profile is sterile before being born; they acquire a tremendous amount during the birthing, and afterwards, from their mother's microbiota, i.e., her vaginal, fecal, skin and breast bacteria. But ultimately all babies develop their own. The development pace is dependent on how the infant is fed, i.e., breast-fed, formula and cow's milk all alter how and what is developed.

Research suggests that by the age of three, the child's microbiota is stable and similar to that of an adult. When we begin to age, the microbiota tends to shift and change again.

Changes in microbiota can cause problems like dysbiosis, or microbial imbalance, which can cause:

- Allergies
- Chronic fatigue syndrome
- Diabetes

- Inflammatory bowel diseases
- Obesity

..and a host of other issues.

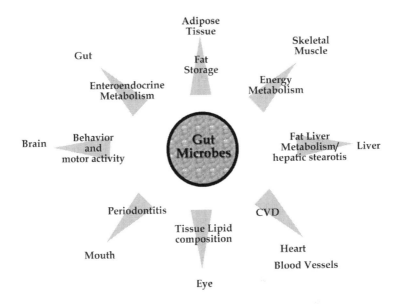

FOUR

What causes the gut to function ineffectively?

If we are designed to have this phenomenal gut system, what can make it become ineffective?

Well, there are all kinds of issues that can contribute to ineffective functioning:

Low pH:

The gut has specific pH levels that vary widely from component to component. On the whole, the North American diet is far too acidic. There are all kinds of contributing factors that cause this acidity but probably one of the worst contributors is sugar. Not only do we eat far too much sugar (the average American sugar intake is 60 lbs. or 28 kg/year!) but also the processed, refined sugar we eat is toxic to the body and brain, and makes us acidic.

Note: Artificial sugar substitutes are just as bad because the body doesn't know the difference.

Poor enzyme activity:

The gut is loaded with enzymes that help us digest our food but most enzymes can only function in a given pH range. When we are too acidic, the enzymes can't function. After a while, the body stops producing them then we are totally reliant on the microbiota to digest our food.

Poor prebiotic:

The microbiota requires its own food to thrive. Their food is what we call the non-soluble type of fibre.

Note: There are two main categories of fibre. The soluble type of fibre is the type that regulates the blood glucose uptake into the liver; the non-soluble type feeds the microbiota and regulates your bowel movements. Each category has several subcategories. Research is now suggesting that there is also a third type of fibre.

The following is a short list on types of fibre and their benefits.

Type of fibre	Soluble/ Insoluble	Food source	Health Benefit
Cellulose, hemiscell-ulose	Insoluble	Nuts, whole wheat, whole grains, bran, seeds, produce skins	Natural laxatives; lowers risk of diverticulitis; helps with weight loss
Inulin oligofructose (digested in the large intestine)	Soluble	Onions, beets or chicory root, byproduct of sugar processing	May support beneficial microflora and immune function
Lignin	Insoluble	Flax, rye, some vegetables	Heart health

Mucilage, beta glucans	Soluble	Herbs like Althea, slippery elm; special mushrooms (cordyceps, reishi, shiitake, maitake) oats, barley, flaxseed, bananas, oranges, carrots	Regulate cholesterols, supports cardio function; prevents diabetes II
Pectin and gums	Mostly soluble	Fruits and berries; seeds	Slows the passage of food through the GIT, allowing for better digestion; regulates cholesterol
Polydextrose	Soluble	Made from dextrose, sorbitol and citric acid	Adds bulk to stool, may prevent constipation
Psyllium	Soluble	Extracted from plantago	Regulates cholesterol and prevents constipation
Resistant starch	Soluble	Found in plant walls: bananas, oatmeal, legumes	Creates sense of fullness – thus helps weight management
Wheat dextrin	Soluble	Extracted from wheat starch	Regulates cholesterol; reduces risk of diabetes

It is also important that when we have good microbiota, these bacteria ferment fibres into short chain fatty acids (SCFA):

- Acetic acid
- Butyric acid
- Propionic acid

In the large intestine these fatty acids have many benefits to the body including:

- The fatty acids noted above supply 50-75% of the energy requirements of the large intestine.
- The production of anti-inflammatories.
- The production of Coenzyme A (used to make our cellular fuel/ATP).

Poor probiotic:

The challenge with taking probiotic supplements is that regardless of how broad a spectrum you take, they usually drop everything into the duodenum – they *do not* all belong there! One nutritional supplement company has developed a patented delivery system that sends different probiotics to different parts of the intestinal tract (see Appendix 2 for more information.)

The following is a short list of beneficial bacteria we find in our gut:

- Lactobacteria
- Bifidobacteria
- Enterococci
- Propionobacteria
- E. coli – the kind found in the lower parts of the intestine use oxygen to clear away the oxygen that may support pathogens. E. coli found elsewhere may cause dysbiosis.
- Peptostreptococci.

These flora produce:

- Anti-biotic substances that can dissolve the membranes of bacteria.
- Anti-fungal substances that can dissolve the membranes of fungus.
- Anti-viral substances that can dissolve the membranes of bacteria.
- They can also chelate heavy metals and other poisons.
- They can trigger our immune response:
  - Neutrophils
  - Macrophages
  - Immune-globulins
  - Interferons
  - Interleukin-1
  - TNF (tumour necrosis factor)
- They also keep the pH near the intestinal wall low, so as to prevent pathogenic bacteria and

other pathogens from moving through the intestinal wall.

- They can also chelate, or bind, to heavy metals and other poisons to eliminate them.

In a healthy adult there should be between 100 billion 1,000 billion healthy bacteria per ml of digestive tract. Unfortunately, in today's civilization, that number can be as low as 5%.

We can also have excessive pathogenic bacteria. When pathogenic bacteria are able to get the upper hand then we have problems. These can include:

- Actinomyces
- Bacterioids
- Clebsielli
- Clostridia
- Corynebacterium
- E. coli (some types)
- Mycobacterium
- Peptococci
- Proteus
- Staphylococci
- Streptococci
- Yeasts
- And many others.

We usually have all of these bacteria but they are kept a given low ratio. In general, the "good bacteria" should make up at least 85% of the gut bacteria. It is when the "bad bacteria" override a healthy ratio and take a dominance that we have problems. For instance, we all have yeast but it is only when the yeast get the upper hand that we have problems.

Many of these pathogenic bacteria will compete for the very nutrients we need. The doctor then tells us to take this supplement, i.e. iron, and we end up feeding it to the pathogens before it ever gets into our system.

Poor diet:

There are all kinds of dietary issues that can cause an imbalance in the microbiota:

- Misuse of alcohol
- Low fruit/vegetable
- High levels of sugars
- High levels of sugary fruits
- High levels of starchy vegetables
- High levels of grains

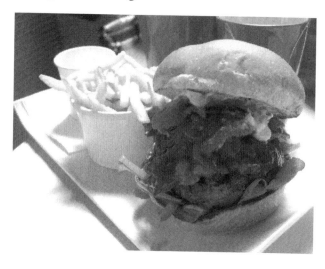

Toxicity:

In our environment today a wide variety of toxicities exist. You have probably heard that we have introduced over 80,000 toxic chemicals into our environment since the Industrial Revolution and that about 80% of those can be found in our homes:

- In our food
- In our water
- In our hygiene products
- In our cleaning products

These toxins include:

- POPs (Persistant Organic Pollutants)
- PCBs (insecticides, herbicides, pesticides, etc.)
- Heavy metal toxicities (mercury, aluminum, arsenic, lead, etc.)

Also, if the gut pathogens are depleting our stores of a given nutrient, i.e., iron, we will be more susceptible to toxicity of another nutrient, such as lead, aluminum or cadmium. Likewise depletion of magnesium allows for the toxicity of aluminum.

Heavy metal toxicity can have the same impact on our microbiota as it does on us.

- They can block the uptake of needed nutrients.
- They can substitute toxic metals for required metals.

- They can alter cell metabolism.
- They can alter enzyme functions.
- They create additional free radicals.

Another toxicity might be copper toxicity. Now, copper toxicity is often due to zinc deficiency. The domino effect then leads to the accumulation of other toxic metals. With copper toxicity we also end up with low levels of hydrochloric acid followed by the decline of important electrolytes like sodium and potassium.

Prolonged stress takes it's toll on the adrenals, which can also cause loss of zinc, as can too much sugar. As zinc goes down, copper goes up and the domino effect noted above continues on.

With depleted levels of hydrochloric acid, we lose our first line of defense for killing pathogens in our food, like salmonella. Low hydrochloric acid can also lead to poor absorption of various nutrients. Low hydrochloric acid can also lead to osteoporosis.

Low Hydrochloric Acid:

As noted above, if the stomach is not producing the required levels of hydrochloric acid, many pathogens get through the stomach and into the intestinal tract, i.e. salmonella. In addition, many nutrients require the hydrochloric acid for absorption, i.e. Vitamin B12, amino acids, calcium and iron. There is also a negative impact on enzyme production in the liver and pancreas when hydrochloric acid is low.

What causes poor hydrochloric acid production? The answer is, low levels of sodium and potassium chloride, which are required to make hydrochloric acid. Copper toxicity, often the result of zinc deficiency, can deplete hydrochloric acid. Zinc deficiency is often the result or prolonged adrenal stress and high sugar intake (which requires the adrenals to regulate blood glucose levels in the blood).

Note: Copper toxicity can result in thyroid impairment, which then makes the body more prone to yeast infections.

Unfortunately, even in our food there can be a disruption between nutrients and bacteria which is subsequently passed on to us.[1]

But the story begins back further than this. If the soil is contaminated the microorganisms in the soil become contaminated, impaired or multi-resistant, all of which can have a huge impact on your gut.[2]

Now let's go a little sideways with this understanding. Research has now demonstrated that human and mice microbiota can transform metals and metalloids into volatile derivatives.[3]

AGEs and free radicals:

AGEs (advanced glycation end-products) can attach to cells and block cell functioning or create cell death, just like a metal toxin. Free radicals steal necessary electrons from other molecules and turn the other molecules into free radicals. Both of these issues impact both gut health and the microbiota.

Overuse of drugs:

Even one dose of anti-biotics can increase yeast and create other conditions in the gut. Anti-biotics not only kill the pathogen bacteria (Note: They do not kill the virus that may be provoking your immune system. Unless you have had a specific test to determine if you have a bacterial or a viral infection, do not take anti-biotics.) but they also indiscriminately kill all the other bacteria in your gut.

Other drugs can also have an impact on your gut microbiota, for instance:

- Hormone elevating drugs like birth control and steroid hormones.
- Anti-inflammatories: NSAIDs will inhibit the growth of healthy bacteria.

FIVE

What happens when the gut isn't functioning properly?

We have already explored what the GI tract does when it functions properly. Obviously, all of these functions do not work effectively when the microbiota is out of balance:

- Food is not effectively digested or absorbed.
- We become deficient in the nutrients that the microbiota make for us.
- Low levels of good bacteria allow the "bad" viruses, mould, yeast, fungi, etc. get out of control.
- The mucosal membrane starts to break down leading to leaky gut syndrome.
- With over 90% of the immune system is in the gut, so our immune system starts to break down.
- We fail to eliminate toxins, bile acids, and cholesterol.
- When the "good" bacteria are deficient, the bad bacteria can utilize our own iron supplies and make us:
  - Anaemic

- o Deplete our red blood supply and oxygen uptake
- o Deplete our energy production
- o Impair detoxification
- These "bad" bacteria can also alter our retention of:
  - o Aluminum, which competes for magnesium. Magnesium is required for over 380 known functions in every cell of the body.
  - o Lead
  - o Cadmium
- We lose the electrolyte balance.
- We find that the water metabolism gets upset.

Other issues start to evolve as well. When the microbiota goes out of balance, inflammatory issues start to evolve:

- Appendicitis
- Colitis
- Crohn's
- IBS

Any of these GI tract inflammatory disorders may have the following symptoms:

- Abdominal pain
- Vomiting
- Diarrhea
- Rectal bleeding

- Internal cramps/spasms

But that isn't all, as a result or alongside of these issues there may also be:

- Allergies
- Anemia
- Arthritis
- Belching
- Bile duct inflammation (causing a variety of liver issues)
- Bloating
- Cell death causing ulcerations (pyoderma gangrenosum)
- Chronic Fatigue Syndrome
- Constipation
- Depression
- Diarrhea
- Dysbiosis – imbalance in the gut microbiota may be the cause or the result of inflammation
- Fatigue
- Fibromyalgia
- Heartburn
- Hemorrhoids
- Hyperactivity, learning and behavioural disorders
- Indigestion
- Joint pain
- Lactose intolerance

- Lowered sex drive
- Mental fog
- Nail fungus
- Skin problems (acne, hives)
- Sugar cravings (including alcohol)
- Thrush
- Weight gain
- Yeast infection

SIX

Poor Liver and Gut Function

This gastrointestinal tube that runs through the body does not operate in isolation, rather in concert with different parts of the body. Science recognizes the liver-gut axis wherein, it is recognized that there is an extensive cross talk with the gut microbioata. The microbiota protects the liver from pathogens and toxins coming down the GIT and the liver protects the vascular/blood lining of the GI tract from toxins inside.

If the microbiota becomes imbalanced, this can lead to intestinal permeability, which then impacts the liver's capacity to carry out over 500 functions. The bacterial and endotoxin translocation then provokes a production of inflammatory cytokines/messengers and other metabolic disorders.

There is an increasing amount of data showing patients with NAFLD (non-alcoholic fatty liver disorder) have increased intestinal permeability/leak gut syndrome and SIBO (small intestinal bacterial overgrowth). In addition, NAFLD also have an overgrowth of some types of bacteria, which may get into the portal blood system and travel to the liver.

The liver is the largest organ of the body and has over 500 functions that support every other system and organ in the body, including the gastrointestinal tract. One of the most well known interactions between the liver and the gut is the liver's constant production of bile. The liver takes cholesterol and converts the cholesterol into bile salts/steroid acids. The main function of bile is to support the formation of micelles.

The bile is stored in the gallbladder until the GIT system is told that fats are coming down the tube. The liver and the gallbladder open the gates and release bile (with the micelles) into the small intestine. The micelles then aid the breakdown of fats in the digestive process.

The membrane lining of the GI tract is also loaded with arteries and veins. The liver plays a huge role in making sure these arteries and veins are clear of various toxins and drugs and pathogens, and loaded with nutrients in order to support the GI tract (and the rest of the body).

When there is dysfunction in the liver because of:

- Cirrhosis – faster transit through the GIT preventing health metabolism and absorption of nutrients.[1]
- High cholesterol – correcting the cholesterol or correcting the microbiota can benefit the other.[2]

- Insulin resistance – high levels of pancreatic insulin secretion can lead to accumulation of liver fat (NAFLD) which can impact on the gut microbiota imbalance and vica versa.[3]
- Gut microbiota plays a role in the development of hepatic steatosis/retention of fats and its progression to non-alcoholic statohepatitis.[4]
- Bile duct inflammation – when the bile ducts that release bile into the small intestine, become inflamed there is a back up that occurs into the liver that can cause liver cirrhosis, liver failure, or liver cancer.

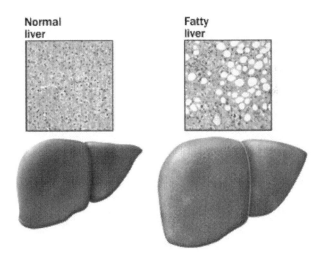

Normal liver

Fatty liver

So it appears that if we want a healthy liver or a healthy gut, we need to take care of both of them, as well as the microbiota.

SEVEN

Poor Pancreatic Function and Gut Flora

The pancreas is not only an endocrine gland that produces hormones like:

- Insulin, which decreases glucose in the blood.
- Glucagon, which increases glucose in the blood.
- Somatostatin, which regulates insulin and glucagon.
- Pancreatic polypeptide, which self regulates the pancreas activities.

It also produces pancreatic juice, which is full of digestive enzymes that empty into the small intestine that help to digest and absorb carbohydrates, fats and lipids.

Research has shown that oral microbiota has an impact on the pancreas.

The gut microbiota impacts the pancreas through the immunological connection, thus the changes in the immune system that the microbiota creates impacts the pancreas. Recent studies indicate that an increase in bacteriodes and a decrease in butyrate-producing bacteria are associated with Type 1 diabetes. Type 1 diabetes is associated with leaky gut syndrome, small intestine inflammation, and food allergies.[1]

But wait, it's not just Type 1 diabetes that is influenced. Research is also showing that the gut microflora also impacts Type 2 diabetes and obesity. Research shows that the gut microbiota impacts:

- Nutrient absorption
- Intestinal transit time
- Bile regulation through the hepatic-gut axis
- Increased cellular uptake of TGs (triglycerides)
- Fatty acid oxidation
- Regulation of low grade inflammation
- Protection of the cellular membrane.

EIGHT

Your Gut and Inflammation

Inflammation has two predominant causes – the immune system and structural damage. Typically, when there is inflammation in the gut it is due to the immune system. We know that the GIT is involved with the following systems:

- Digestive system.
- Immune system, to protect it.
- Hormone/endocrine, to talk to the brain, the liver and the pancreas to let them know what is required from them.
- Neurological system, to stimulate or inhibit organs and muscles when necessary.
- Cardiovascular system, to bring nutrients and oxygen through the blood and to remove toxins and excesses.
- Hepatic system, to bring in bile/bile salts to break down the fats.
- Pancreatic system, to bring in enzymes for digestion.
- Enzymes, released from inside of the intestinal tract and brought in from organs outside of the tract, i.e. pancreas.

- Microbiota, to help with digestion, to support the immune system, and to provide nutrients that we require.

If there is a problem with any one of these systems, we may end up with an inflammatory problem. Some of the gut inflammatory conditions are:

Inflammatory bowel disorders:

IBD – Inflammatory bowel disease

- UC – ulcerative colitis – affects the mucosal lining of the gut.
- Crohn's disease – can affects any part of the gut.
- Collagenous colitis – affects the colon.
- Lymphocytic colitis – chronic non-bloody watery diarrhea.
- Ischaemic colitis – inflammation/injury results from inadequate blood supply.
- Diversion colitis – inflammation condition as a result of surgery.
- Beheet's disease – an immune disorder that effects the mucous membrane.
- Indeterminate colitis.

Any of these disorders may cause or may be the cause of:

- IBS – irritable bowel syndrome – alteration in bowel movements

- Probiotic disruption – there are over 1000 different types of bacteria in the gut.
- Constipation
- Diarrhea
- Leaky gut syndrome
- Neurological disorders:
  o Depression
  o Bipolar
  o Autism
  o Schizophrenia
  o Parkinson's
  o Alzheimer's
- Adrenal disorders
- Liver disorders
- Metabolic disorders
- Allergies
- Chronic Fatigue Syndrome
- Toxicities, and much more.

How does inflammation in the gut evolve? There are a number of causes of gut inflammation:

Lack of nutrienst or damaging nutrients:

- AGEs (Advanced Glycation Endproducts) created when sugar combines with either fats or proteins without enzyme direction.
  o This can happen while we are cooking.
  o This can happen in our gut with excess sugars.

Excess free radicals:

- Caused by poor nutrients; excess sugars; excess toxins.

Nutrient deficient foods:

- Pasteurized foods
- Microwaved foods
- Processed foods
- Fast foods
- GMOs (genetically modified organisms)

Excess toxins:

- Environmental toxins
- Pharmaceutical toxins
- Vaccinations
- Anti-biotics
- Anti-depressants
- NSAIDs
- Aspirin
- Ibuprofen
- Arthritic prescriptions
- Naproxen
- Anti cancer treatments
- Chemotherapy
- Radiation therapy
- Corticosteroids
- POPs (persistent organic pollutants)

- PCBs (insecticides, pesticides, herbicides, etc.)
- Toxins found in our cleaning products:
  - Personal hygiene
  - Home hygiene
  - Laundry

Depleted immune system:

- Caused by other disorders/diseases/dysfunctions in the system.
- Caused by depleted levels of glutathione required by the immune system to both develop and respond as well as to regulate balances between different immune factors, for instance T1 and T2.
- Depleted nutrients required by the immune system.

Depleted microbiota:

- Depleted nutrients
- Excess toxins
- Bowel issues, i.e. diarrhea
- Inflammation
- Depleted immune system

Are you starting to understand how inter-reactive, inter-dependent, inter-dynamic these systems are?

Unfortunately, western conventional medicine has lost an understanding of this. Western conventional medicine has become so reductionist it has lost its ability to work effectively with this very dynamic interactive system. With any given diagnosis, or profile of symptoms, there can be a multitude of causes; causes that overlap, causes that sequentially evolve, and causes that can be the result of other causes.

Very often we find that given patterns of health issues co-exist. For instance, if you are eating a fast food diet with loads of detrimental sugars and detrimental fats, drinking sodas loaded with sugars and toxins, eating microwaved diners and popcorn, all full of calories but depleted of nutrients, you are going to have a number of problems evolve in the body.

Note: Some people are sensitive to even a small amount of these foods, while others can withstand a small amount but over a prolonged period of time. Others can handle a lot of it before they start experiencing problems.

The challenge is, the problems don't usually occur immediately. The system is loaded with all kinds of compensatory systems and feedback loops. The interactive, inter-dynamic compilation of systems, in the human body, keeps compensating and compensating until it just cannot compensate any longer. When we are out of compensatory mechanisms, we start to see the symptoms and problems. By this time, we have:

- Inflammation in the gut.
- A depleted microbiota – of which you are probably not aware.
- A non-alcoholic fatty liver – of which you are not aware.
- Depleted glutathione – of which you are not aware.
- Depleted minerals – of which you are not aware.
- Adrenal issues – of which you are not aware.
- Syndrome X/metabolic syndrome or diabetes – of which you are not aware.
- Cardiovascular issues – of which you are not aware.
- Allergies – of which you may not be aware since too narrow a spectrum of bacteria leads to allergies.
- Foggy brain syndrome.
- A lack of energy.
- Feeling overwhelmed.

Whichever symptom stands out the most for you, you tell the MD about. He or she prescribes a drug to deal with that particular symptom but the whole diversity of underlying issues continues to move further and further out of balance.

The drugs may or may not relieve the symptoms but will further deplete the body of nutrients.

We need to take care of the underlying problems before we have major issues. Taking care of the inflammatory/immune/microbiota in the gut is often the first place to start.

NINE

Connection between Gut Disorders and Neurological Disorders.

As we noted in Chapter Two, when the gut is not functioning effectively all systems can be affected. Let's look at a few other issues.

The brain is made up of:

- Millions of neurons.
- With a huge number that have extensions/axons that travel down the spinal cord and out through the body.
- Even more neurotransmitters: monoamines, peptides, etc.
- Lots of hormones.
- Various components: hippocampus, hypothalamus
- Various glands such as pituitary and pineal.
- Various systems – motor, limbic, visual, etc.
- Fluids like blood, lymph, cerebral spinal fluid

The brain is made up of about 70 fats, uses 20% of the body's oxygen, and about 50% of the body's blood glucose. Okay, so the brain needs a lot of nutrients.

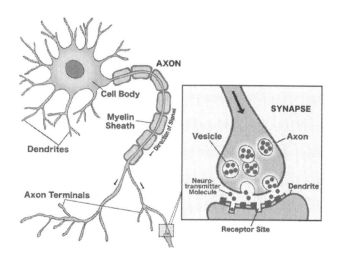

Those nutrients have to initially come from our dietary intake into the gut and from the gut into the rest of the body.

Excess or deficiency in any of the following nutrients can disrupt brain function:

- Minerals:
  - Magnesium
  - Iron
  - Zinc
  - Copper
  - Manganese
- Anti-oxidants:
  - Glutathione
  - Superoxide dismutase
- Vitamins:
  - Vitamin A
  - Vitamin B1, B3, B5, B6 B9, B12

- o Vitamin C
- Fats:
  - o ALA
  - o DHA
  - o EPA
  - o Choline, needed to make Acetylcholine
- Amino acids: (the base structures for neurotransmitters.
  - o Glutamate
  - o Phenylalanine, needed for norepinephrine and dopamine
  - o Tyrosine (energizing effect) needed for norepinephrine and dopamine, thyroid hormones T3 and T4 also needed for the brain
  - o Tryptophan (calming effect) needed for serotonin, 5HTP.

Consequently, if the gut is *not* functioning effectively, and we are not absorbing these nutrients or the nutrients required to make these compounds then our brain is at a disadvantage and a number of problems can develop. Research is now showing that there is not only a major gut-brain axis/communication, which is a bidirectional communication, but that there is also a microbiata-gut-brain axis. However, we are only just beginning to understand the complexities involved.

Some theories suggest that the microbiota may affect the brain through the mucosal immune system. I would suggest that there are a variety of mechanisms through which the gut can have an impact on the brain. For instance:

- The microbiota may have a direct impact on the host DNA which impacts on the brain.
- The microbiota may have an indirect impact on the host DNA through the by-products that result from the ingestion/fermentation of the fibre in the gut, which can cross the blood/brain barrier.
- The microbiota may impact the brain through the immune system:
  o Activation of different inflammatory mechanisms.
  o Activitation of different T cells.
  o Given species can cause specific issues:
    ▪ Citrobacter rodentium – impact on learning and memory; anxiety.
    ▪ Mycobacterium bovis – impacts depression, anxiety and cognitive dysfunction.
    ▪ Trichuris muris – causes anxiety.[1]
- The microbiota may impact the brain when they are diminished and:
  o Leak guy syndrome develops.
  o Required nutrients are taken from the host by the pathogen.
- That some microbiota can affect the brain through the vagus nerve.[2]

- We already know that when various microbiota species are dominant over others, a huge number of other issues can occur from depression and anxiety to weight issues.

Further, if the probiotics in the gut are not functioning effectively, we can experience issues with:

1) Depression
2) Bipolar
3) Schizophrenia
4) Parkinson's
5) Alzheimer's
6) Visual issues
7) Motor issues
8) Sensory issues

And many more. Let's look at a few of these issues.

Depression:

Did you know that research has shown that Borrelia burgdorferi/Lyme disease causes depression in up to two-thirds of all cases, as well as:

- Obsessive-compulsive disorder
- Panic disorders and phobias
- Dementia
- Non-Hodgkin lymphomas
- Arthritis
- Arrhythmia
- Arthralgia
- Meningitis

- Facial nerve palsy.[3,4]

Just as an aside, did you know that there is about an 80% correlation between people with depression and people suffering from constipation? Does the constipation cause depression? Or does depression cause constipation? Or is it a third factor that causes both? Or perhaps an evolution of issues...

For instance:

- Hypothyroidism is related to both depression and constipation.
- Anti-depressants (SSRIs and Tricyclics) can cause constipation. (Note: Low serotonin levels have never been proven to cause depression. Regulating serotonin has never been proven to resolve depression, and you make most of the serotonin in your gut – not your brain!)
- Irritable bowel syndrome (often caused by gut dysbiosis/imbalance in the microbiota) is closely linked to depression.
- Antacids (taken for heartburn) prevent the stomach from making the hydrochloric acid, which kills pathogens. So now the pathogens make it through and cause constipation – which is linked with depression. (Note: When you take antacids for heartburn, the stomach initially becomes more alkaline and then responds by making even more hydrochloric acid – not a good move. Further, the antacids

often contain aluminum therefore contributing to metal toxicity.)

- High blood pressure medications (calcium channel blockers or diuretics) can cause constipation. High blood pressure and depression are also related. Anxiety can cause depression.
- Anti-histamines can cause constipation and can cause depression.
- Diets high in cheese and other high fat/low fibre foods can cause constipation and there is a link between high fat foods and depression.[5]

And the list goes on. But the gut-brain connection doesn't just have an impact on depression. Let's look at another issue – Alzheimer's.

Alzheimer's Disease:

We think of Alzheimer's, like depression, as a brain issue but there are lots of issues that may cause Alzheimer's. For instance:

- The oldest theory concerning the cause of Alzheimer's has to do with the body's capacity to make a neurotransmitter called acetylcholine but the theory has lost most of its support.
- Another theory concerned amyloidosis – beta amyloid deposits; subsequent theories have looked at other amyloid issues.

- The tau hypothesis addresses a tau protein that forms neurofibrillary/fibrin tangles inside of neurons.
- Herpes simplex has also been identified as a causative factor.
- Low levels of glutathione allowing for oxidative stress and inflammation.
- Changes in the immune cells have also been identified in Alzheimer's[,6] but this may be a reflection of low levels of glutathione, in consideration of the fact that immune cells require glutathione to both develop and function.
- Metal toxicities like aluminum, chloride, iron and copper.[7]

Research also shows that the microbiota affects the lipid metabolism in the host. We said earlier that the brain is made up of 70% fats, which provide:

- Structure
- Transport mechanisms
- Axon insulation
- Energy.

So if there is a problem with lipid/fat metabolism or fatty acid metabolism, the brain is going to have difficulties. One of the possible mechanisms for disrupting lipid/fat metabolism is in the gut. Research results indicate that several different types of bacteria are involved in the metabolism of lipids/fats in the body.[8] These include:

- Firmicutes
- Actinobacteria
- Proteobacteria

If the good healthy fats that the body requires don't get metabolized, the brain suffers.

We find similar issues with a wide variety of neurological disorders from schizophrenia to Parkinson's to Alzheimer's. As we can see, there is a definite connection between the gut and the brain.

TEN

Connection between Gut Disorders and Cardiovascular Disorders.

Imbalance in the gut microbiota can also be an environmental risk factor for cardiovascular problems. That means anything from the heart to the blood vessels (both arteries and veins) to the lungs, liver and kidneys that all play a major role in the blood cleaning/exchange process.

Apparently, the gut microbiota are involved in converting choline (a molecule found in eggs, beef and pork) to trimethylamine. Lots of big words...so let's try to make it simple:

We make phosphatidylcholine (important for the brain and the cell membranes). The gut bacteria take the choline out of the phosphatidylcholine (using hydrolysis) then convert the choline to trimethylamine. Trimethylamine then gets converted in the liver to TMAO, which then goes into the blood. TMAO alters cholesterol metabolism in the gut, liver and arterial walls. When TMAO is present, more cholesterol is deposited into the arterial walls and other locations.[1]

Now cholesterol is very important to our whole system. We need cholesterol for the following reasons:

- Outer rim of the cell – required to regulate what goes in and out of the cell.
- Bile – breaks down the fats that you digest and allows you to absorb the good fats.
- Hormones – all the steroid hormones like testosterone, estrogen, cortisol, aldosterone.
- Vitamin D – required to make Vitamin D.
- Insulation – the neurons in the brain require proper insulation to work and they need fat.
- Absorption of fat based vitamins: A, D, E, K.
- Acts as an anti-oxidant.
- Contributes to bone formation – they would be hollow and brittle without it.
- Cholesterol plaque is there to protect damaged arteries. A clogged artery is better than a ruptured one.
- Oxidation of cholesterol is the first step by which cholesterol transforms into Vitamin D3.
- Cholesterol sulphate deficiency leads to glucose intolerance.

We also have to take into consideration that there are many different types of cholesterol:

- HDL 2a and 2b, want to be high – extracts fats from arterial walls and prevents fats from adhering to the walls.

- HDL 3 – want to be lower than HDL 2.
- LDL A – large and buoyant LDL. This is what you want.
- LDL B – predominantly small and dense LDL. You don't want this as it is implicated in diabetes, high blood pressure, and arteriosclerosis.
- LDL mixed.
- LDL R – associated with a bad diet.
- LDL a – a good inflammatory marker.
- IDL – similar to an LDL but without the TG, transports TG fats and cholesterols and can promote growth of atheroma.
- Lp(a) Lipoprotein consists of an LDL-like particle and controlled genetically, kidney function important for clearing it.
- VLDL 1,2 – very large and transports TGs to adipose and muscle.

So while the gut microbiata alter cholesterol and the deposits of cholesterol, further studies are required concerning:

- The type of cholesterol.
- The role of cholesterol in the arterial wall, i.e. is it patching up a leaky artery or is it just causing problems.
- This is a huge conflict between conventional and traditional and alternative medicines. Conventional medicine practitioners think

cholesterol is causing the problem, whereas traditional medicine practitioners believe that the cholesterol is like a firefighter at the scene of a fire. Whether it is a slow leak or inflammation of the blood vessel, cholesterol is there to help the problem.

- However, even if the cholesterol is the firefighter at the scene of the fire, it the cholesterol that continues to accumulate at the site. it will slow down the flow of blood and will cause a problem.

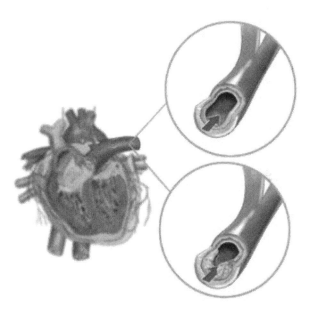

While most of the research to date connecting the gut microbiota and the cardiovascular system has focused on the ability of the microbes to metabolize cholesterol, other problems can also occur.

For instance, what happens when toxins from the gut leak into the blood system? What if the immune system in the gut breaks down and pathogens leak into the blood? What if inflammation in the gut provokes:

- Atherosclerosis
- Myopathies
- Phlebitis
- Thrombosis
- Vasculitis?

Again, we need the gut to provide nutrients for the rest of the body and to protect the rest of the body from toxins and pathogens.

ELEVEN

Connection between Gut Disorders and
Weight Issues.

There are also connections between weight issues and activities in the gut. Some are associated with the microbiota while are not. The connection is usually associated with the diversity and/or the dominance of difference bacteria.

For instance, studies both in humans and in mice have shown a connection between both a lower diversity in the microbes and/or a decreased level in Bacteroidetes with obesity.[2,3]

Conversely, Fredrik Backhed showed that if the microbiota shuts down the FIAF (fasting induced adipose factor) gene then a series of events occurred (involving increased glucose uptake in the small intestine and fermentation of carbohydrates into short chain fatty acids in the large intestine) wherein the mice were protected from an obesity-induced diet.[4]

On the other hand, inflammation in the gut can also be an issue. For instance, in another study researchers found that those subjects who ate just the McDonald's breakfast had increased blood levels of a molecule called endotoxin. This molecule comes from the outer walls of certain bacteria. When our bodies perceive endotoxin, the immune system responds with inflammation.

There is evidence indicating the gut microbiota can extract calories from ingested foods and help to store in the host fat cells for later use.[1]

Wow! You mean they are storing calories in my fat cells, for their future use?

Let's take this a step further. Scientists looked at two groups of mice. One group of mice had a 40% higher ratio of body fat, even though they were fed less than their counterparts. They took the gut microbiota from the first group and transplanted it into a second group of mice. The second group of mice increased their body weight by 60% in 2 weeks. There was no difference in food consumption or energy expenditure/exercise. But there was a 60% increase in weight!

The second group of mice not only had an increase in body fat but, in addition, they:

- Developed insulin resistance.
- Adipocyte hypertrophy (excess body fat)
- Increased levels of blood glucose.
- Increased levels of circulating leptin (a hormone that stimulates the sense of hunger and a variety of other issues).[5]

All because their gut bacteria was changed!

As pointed out in my book: *Managing Your Weight: Why your body may be working against you and what you can do about it,* there are lots of confounding issues that play into weight metabolism. Simply looking at diet and metabolism just don't cut it. From the pH of the gut to the enzymes in the gut, to the bacteria in the gut, these are just a few of the issues that should be considered.

There is a multitude of other issues in the gut that may also play a role in weight management. For instance, Dr. Dandona claims that the real issue is inflammation. When doing a study of people who ate "a simple McDonald's meal that seems harmless enough", he found a dramatic inflammatory effect that lasted for hours.[6]

Inflammation didn't simply result from the McDonald's breakfast, rather in reaction to what the gut bacteria did with it. The gut bacteria inflammation issue is not only a key to weight gain but also to insulin resistance, diabetes, and a host of other conditions.

PART III

TWELVE

How to Effectively Support Your Gut

There is a variety of ways to effectively support your gut, which include:

- Foods to eat
- Foods to avoid
- Supplements to take.

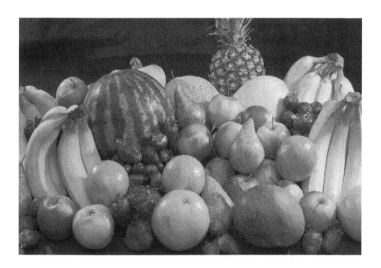

Foods to eat:

When effectively feeding the gut (and the rest of your body), the body obviously needs good healthy foods. Although the body requires nutrients to do millions of functions, here we are specifically looking at the nutrients it requires to support gut functions. In particular, we are looking at the requirements of the following processes:

- Anti-inflammatory foods
- Immune supporting foods
- Microbiota supporting foods.

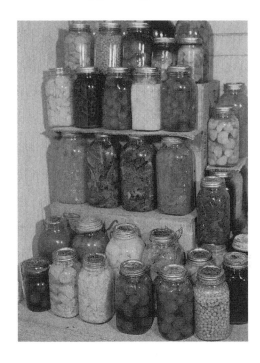

So, let's start with the basics that most people know already:

- Eat whole organic foods.
- Eat less meat and eat organic meat.

- Steam vegetables – provokes the enzymes and doesn't lose the nutrients.
- Fermented foods:
- Chinese pickles
- Fermented bean paste
- Fish sauce
- Kefir
- Kimchi
- Miso
- Sauerkraut
- Shrimp paste
- Sinki

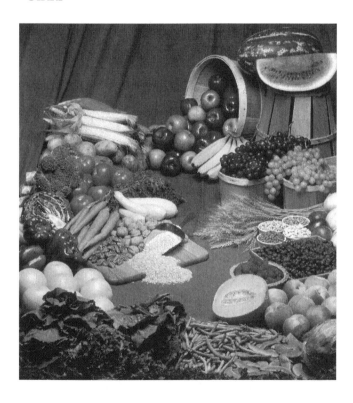

- Sourdough
- Soy sauce
- Tapai
- Worcestershire sauce
- Yogurt

Fibrous foods (to feed the bacteria):

- Almonds
- Apples
- Artichokes
- Avocados
- Barley
- Beans: black, white, kidney, garbanzo
- Broccoli
- Corn
- Edamame (immature soybeans – make sure they are not GMO)
- Lentils
- Oatmeal (organic, steel cut oats)
- Pears (with peel)
- Pees
- Raspberries
- Rice: brown (2 or less servings decreases diabetes; 5 or more increases risk of diabetes)
- White beans

Healthy fats:

- Avocados
- Camelina oil

- Chia
- Coconut
- Grape seed oil
- Macadamia nuts
- Oils: nut, grain and seed oils are good for you, but Olive oil is of no value 6 months after it has been processed)
- Seeds: flax, hemp or chia/salba
- Shea butter

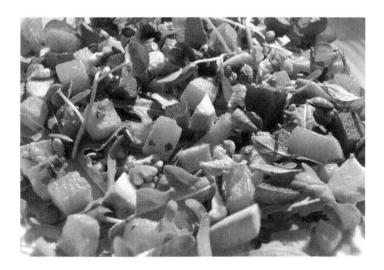

If you need to eat breads, choose:

- Sourdough (fermented)
- German Rye (anti-carcinogenic)
- Sprouted (sprouting provokes the enzymes)

Also:

- Honey (There is a variety of non-pasteurized honeys that are very good for you.)
- Apple Cider vinegar (with a good "mother").
- Whole lemons (inner and outer rinds, seeds, the whole thing).

Anti-inflammatory foods:

- Berries: blueberries, raspberries, strawberries (make sure they are organic
- Green leafed vegetables: kale, spinach
- Whole grains: quinoa, barley, steel cut oats
- Healthy oils: krill, salmon, cod liver
- Healthy fish: salmon, tuna, sardines

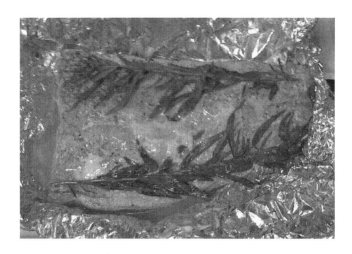

Foods to avoid:

- GMOs (genetically modified organisms).

- NON-organic foods sprayed with pesticides, insecticides, etc.
- Processed foods (canned, packaged, pre-prepared).
- Microwaved foods (including microwaved popcorn; eliminates the nutrients)
- Pasteurized foods (eliminates the nutrients)
- Fast foods (full of bad fats and lack nutrients)
- White sugars:
- Baking: breads, cakes, pies, cookies
- Junk food: chocolate bars, candies, ice cream, milk shakes, gum
- Drinks: sodas, store bought juice, drink powders
- Dried fruit, canned fruit: apples, dates, apricots, raisins, figs, etc.

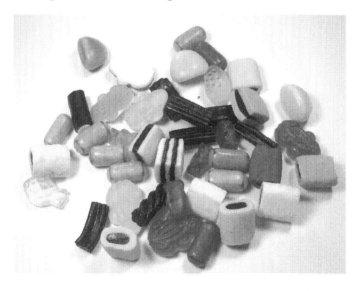

- Spreads: jams, preserves,
- Cereals: boxed cereals, cereal bars, granola, oatmeal packages
- Condiments: ketchup, salad dressings
- Artificial sugars (just as toxic to the body and brain as white sugar):
  o Acesulfame-K
  o Aspartame
  o NutraSweet
  o Saccharin
  o Sucralose
- Flours:
- White flour
- Whole-wheat flour (Two slices of whole wheat bread is equivalent to a snickers bar.)
- Pasta
- Salted foods: potato chips, peanuts,

Know what your allergies are. During the healing process, make sure you eliminate the allergen foods, i.e. dairy or gluten.

Supplements to take:

- Probiotics: Be careful of the probiotic that you take. You not only want a good breadth of good bacteria, but you also want a good delivery system. If all of the probiotic is dropped in the duodenum of the small intestine – you will lose most of it. You want a probiotic that delivers different probiotics to different segments of the intestinal tract.

- Fibre: Probiotics need to feed on their food. They also change the fibre into nutrients we need. If you cannot get sufficient fibre in your diet, then take some in a supplement.

- Glutathione: Some products work, some don't.

Effective:

- We can products that turn on the DNA tools (mRNA) that make the glutathione. (See Appendix 2 for more information.)

- We can take products that provide the ingredients to make the GSH component of the glutathione complex. (See Appendix 2 for more information.)

- We can take clinical supplements that provide the ingredients to make all 8 glutathione components in the glutathione complex.

- We can take Nano-sized glutathione in a phosphotidyalcholine transport mechanism that pushes through the cell membrane and delivers the glutathione to the cell.

Ineffective:

- We can individual products that provide some of the nutrients to make glutathione:

- NAC – N-acetyl-choline.

- Whey products – have to take an awful lot to get sufficient cysteine.

- Whole glutathione (GSH) breaks down in the GIT. Even if it didn't, there are no transport mechanisms to absorb it into the cells so it creates expensive bowel movements.

- We can get glutathione injections. The problem is that it will fill the blood with glutathione which will then trigger feedback loops in the cells which will then stop making glutathione

For more information about all the different functions of glutathione see Appendix 1 and 2.

   o Transfer Factor: there are 8 different types of known transfer factor in the body and 6 of those are in the gut. When there are problems in the gut/body/brain very often we require transfer factors to "reprogram" the immune system in the gut in order to heal.

- For more information: Go to Appendix 2.

   o 5 herb formulation that turns on the DNA genes that make anti-oxidants:
      o Glutathione
      o Super oxide dismutase
      o Catalase

As well as:

- The inflammatory system
- The anti-fibrosis system
  (For more information, go to Appendix 2.)

- Minerals: Most of us are deficient in various minerals, such as magnesium. The soils are depleted so the plants and animals are depleted, so we are depleted. We need magnesium for over 380 known basic cell functions but we need to take a good source of magnesium, like ionic citrate magnesium, which has a high bioavailability or absorption and usability ration.

The very drugs that we take to eliminate symptoms may be adding to the underlying problems:

- Drugs tend to deplete the body of the very nutrients the body requires to heal.
- Drugs depend on the body to metabolize them and eliminate them, thus further depleting the nutrients.
- Drugs usually are not aimed at solving the problem, only covering up or eliminating the perceived symptoms.

Exercise adds the body's capacity to function, however…

- Too much exercise depletes the body's nutrients, i.e. glutathione.

- Too little exercise enables the pathogens, toxins, etc. to accumulate and cause more damage.

Perhaps one of the best things you might do for yourself is to find a good health practitioner.

Note: MDs are trained to be symptom managers. They have virtually no training in the nutrients the body requires or what the body does with the nutrients. They are trained in pharmaceutical protocols, not in all the different types of toxicities or how to eliminate them.

A good health practitioner is trained in recognizing what symptoms indicate:

- Allergies
- Toxins
- Deficiencies

They are trained in how to eliminate the underlying cause as opposed to simply treating the symptoms.

Here's to your healthy journey.

Appendix 1

WHAT DO YOU KNOW ABOUT GLUTATHIONE?

Master Anti-oxidant

- Endogenous – made inside of the cell
- Re-stabilizes itself and all other anti-oxidants
- Deals with all 6 categories of free radicals
- Works inside cell; in cell membrane; and outside of cell

Detoxification

- Major component of Phase II in liver detox
- Major component of all cellular detoxification

Inflammation

- Major component of healthy inflammation resolution

Hormone regulation

- Involved either directly or indirectly with all hormones in the body

Cellular Energy

- Cellular energy is provided by the ATP; created by the mitochondria – GSH is the only known molecule that protects the mitochondria

Prostaglandin synthesis:

- vasodilation/constriction of arteries

Nitric oxide regulation:

- hormones, vasodilation, immune system,

DNA

- Protects DNA from going sideways; involved in both or elimination of abnormal DNA

- also required in protein synthesis

Cellular transport

- Required for most amino acid transportation in the cells

Anti-aging

- Involved, like other anti-oxidants, in preventing telomere breakdown but also the only known molecule that can provoke telomere creation

Calcium movement

- Required for regulation of Calcium movement (gating of cardio cell function)

Respiratory

- 40% required in RBC to both pick up/release both O2 and CO2

Immune System

- Lymphocytes, i.e. T cells, B cells, cacrophages, TNF, NK, ets. All require about 62% to both develop and to function.

- Regulation balance between defferent types of immune cellse, i.e. T1 and T2.

What destroys glutathione:

- Age
- Pollution
- Genetic abnormalities
- Stress
- Overuse of drugs
- Infections
- Injuries
- Radiation
- Poor diet
- Too much sun
- Lack of hydration
- Exercising past a sweat
- Poor sleeping habits
- Pesticides and certain food additives
- Drugs (alcohol, tobacco, legal and illegal drugs)

Appendix 2:

To learn more about or purchase products please visit Dr. Holly's website at www.choicesunlimited.ca.

Tables

Table of Hormones:
http://users.rcn.com/jkimball.ma.ultranet/BiologyP
ages/H/HormoneTable.html

Table of Neurotransmitters:
http://en.wikipedia.org/wiki/Neurotransmitters

References:

Alisi, Anna, et al. Causative role of gut microbiota in non-alcoholic fatty liver disease pathogenesis. http://www.frontiersin.org/Cellular_and_Infection_Microbiology/10.3389/fcimb.2012.00132/full

Backhed, Fredrik. Mechanisms underlying the resistance to diet-induced obesity in germ free mice. Proc Natl Acad Sci U S A. 2007 January 16; 104(3): 979-984.

Bercik, Premsyl. The mirobiota – gut – brain axis: learning from intestinal bacteria? http://gut.bmj.com/content/60/3/288.extract

Bested, Alison et al. Gut Pathogens. http://www.gutpathogens.com/content/5/1/5

Bransfield, Robert, MD. Sex and Lyme Disease. http://www.mentalhealthandillness.com/Articles/S exAndLymeDisease.htm

Caliz, Joan, et al. Emerging resistant microbiota from an acidic soil exposed to toxicity of Cr, Cd and Pb is mainly influenced by the bioavailability of these metals.

http://link.springer.com/article/10.1007%2Fs11368-012-0609-7

Collins, Stephen, MB.BS. FRCPC. Intestinal Microbiota and the Brain-Gut Axis. http://hstalks.com/main/view_talk.php?t=2103andr=609andj=756andc=252

DeBaise, J, et al. Gut microbiota and its possible relationship with obesity. Mayo Clinic Proceedings. Vol. 83, Issue 4, Pages 460-469, April 2008

Gielda, Lindsay, et al. Zinc competition among the Intestinal Microbiota. http://mbio.asm.org/content/3/4/e00171-12.full

Karlsen, S, et al. Small intestinal transit in patients with liver cirrhosis and portal hypertension: a descriptive study. http://www.ncbi.nlm.nih.gov/pubmed/23216853

Lahti, L, et al. Associations between the human intestinal microbiota, Lactobacillus rhamnosus GG and serum lipids indicated by integrated analysis of high-throughput proliling data. http://www.ncbi.nlm.nih.gov/pubmed/23638368

Ley R. E., Turnbaugh P. J., Klein S., Gordon J. I. 2006. Microbial ecology: human gut microbes associated with obesity. Nature. 444: 1022–1023.

Martorana, Adriana et al. Immunosenescence, Inflammation and Alzheimer's disease.

http://www.longevityandhealthspan.com/content/1/1/8

Michalke, Klaus et al. Role of Intestinal Microbiota in Transformation of Bismuth and other metals and metalloids into volatile methyl and hydride derivatives in humans and mice. http://aem.asm.org/content/74/10/3069.full.pdf

Musso, Giovanni, et al. Interactions between gut microbiota and host metabolism predisposing to obesity and diabetes. http://www.annualreviews.org/doi/full/10.1146/annurev-med-012510-175505

Vaarala, Outi. Gut microbiota and type 1 diabetes. Found in: https://www.soc-bdr.org/orderforms/content/rds/special_issues/immunology_of_type_1_diabetes/early_view_articles/gut_microbiota_and_type_1_diabetes/index_en.html

Vajro, P, et al. Microbiota and gut-liver axis: their influences on obesity and obesity-related liver disease. http://www.ncbi.nlm.nih.gov/pubmed/23287807

Velasquez-Manoff, Moises. Are Happy Gut Bacteria Key to Weight Loss? http://www.motherjones.com/environment/2013/04/gut-microbiome-bacteria-weight-loss

A new target in fighting brain disease: Metals. Found in:

http://online.wsj.com/article/SB10001424052970204
74090457719290107261l524.html

Everything you always wanted to know about the
Gut microbiota.
http://www.gutmicrobiotawatch.org/gut-
microbiota-info/

Gut Flora and Metal.
http://www.tvernonlac.com/gutflora.html

Link examined between high fat diet and depression.
http://www.recoveryranch.com/articles/news/high
-fat-food-depression/

Lyme Disease Worldwide Support. Found in:
http://www.lyme.ws/lyme-disease-and-mental-
illness/

Role of Intestinal microbiota in transformation of
bismuth and other metals and metalloids into volatile
methyl and hydride derivatives in humans and mice.
http://aem.asm.org/content/74/10/3069.full.pdf

Trimethylamine N-oxide.
http://en.wikipedia.org/wiki/TMAO#Health_issues

References and Quotes:

Chapter 3

1 Gut Flora and Metal.
http://www.tvernonlac.com/gutflora.html

[2] DeBaise, J, et al. Gut microbiota and its possible relationship with obesity. Mayo Clinic Proceedings. Vol. 83, Issue 4, Pages 460-469, April 2008

[3] DeBaise, J, et al. Gut microbiota and its possible relationship with obesity. Mayo Clinic Proceedings. Vol. 83, Issue 4, Pages 460-469, April 2008

Chapter 4

[1] Gielda, Lindsay, et al. Zinc competition among the Intestinal Microbiota.
http://mbio.asm.org/content/3/4/e00171-12.full

[2] Caliz, Joan, et al. Emerging resistant microbiota from an acidic soil exposed to toxicity of Cr, Cd and Pb is mainly influenced by the bioavailability of these metals.
http://link.springer.com/article/10.1007%2Fs11368-012-0609-7

[3] Role of Intestinal microbiota in transformation of bismuth and other metals and metalloids into volatile methyl and hydride derivatives in humans and mice.
http://aem.asm.org/content/74/10/3069.full.pdf

Chapter 6

[1] Karlsen, S, et al. Small intestinal transit in patients with liver cirrhosis and portal hypertension: a descriptive study. Found in:
http://www.ncbi.nlm.nih.gov/pubmed/23216853

[2] Alisi, Anna, et al. Causative role of gut microbiota in non-alcoholic fatty liver disease pathogenesis.

http://www.frontiersin.org/Cellular_and_Infection_
Microbiology/10.3389/fcimb.2012.00132/full

[3] Alisi, Anna, et al. Causative role of gut microbiota
in non-alcoholic fatty liver disease pathogenesis.
Found in:
http://www.frontiersin.org/Cellular_and_Infection_
Microbiology/10.3389/fcimb.2012.00132/full

[4] Vajro, P, et al. Microbiota and gut-liver axis: their
influences on obesity and obesity-related liver
disease. Found in:
http://www.ncbi.nlm.nih.gov/pubmed/23287807

Chapter 7

[1] Vaarala, Outi. Gut microbiota and type 1 diabetes.
https://www.soc-
bdr.org/orderforms/content/rds/special_issues/im
munology_of_type_1_diabetes/early_view_articles/g
ut_microbiota_and_type_1_diabetes/index_en.html

Chapter 8

[1] Bercik, Premsyl. The mirobiota – gut – brain axis:
learning from intestinal bacteria?
http://gut.bmj.com/content/60/3/288.extract

[2] Collins, Stephen, MB.BS. FRCPC. Intestional
Microbiota and the Brain-Gut Axis.
http://hstalks.com/main/view_talk.php?t=2103andr
=609andj=756andc=252

[3]Bransfield, Robert, MD. Sex and Lyme Disease. http://www.mentalhealthandillness.com/Articles/SexAndLymeDisease.htm

[4]Lyme Disease Worldwide Support. http://www.lyme.ws/lyme-disease-and-mental-illness/

[5]Link examined between high fat diet and depression. http://www.recoveryranch.com/articles/news/high-fat-food-depression/

[6]Martorana, Adriana et al. Immunosenescence, Inflammation and Alzheimer's disease. http://www.longevityandhealthspan.com/content/1/1/8

[7]A new target in fighting brain disease: Metals. http://online.wsj.com/article/SB10001424052970204740904577192901072611524.html

[8]Lahti, L, et al. Associations between the human intestinal microbiota, Lactobacillus rhamnosus GG and serum lipids indicated by integrated analysis of high-throughput proliling data. http://www.ncbi.nlm.nih.gov/pubmed/23638368

Chapter 9

[1] Trimethylamine N-oxide. http://en.wikipedia.org/wiki/TMAO#Health_issues

Chapter 10

[1]Ley R. E., Turnbaugh P. J., Klein S., Gordon J. I. 2006. Microbial ecology: human gut microbes associated with obesity. Nature. 444: 1022–1023.

[2]Ley R. E., Turnbaugh P. J., Klein S., Gordon J. I. 2006. Microbial ecology: human gut microbes associated with obesity. Nature. 444: 1022–1023.

[3]Backhed, Fredrik. Mechanisms underlying the resistance to diet-induced obesity in germ free mice. Proc Natl Acad Sci U S A. 2007 January 16; 104(3): 979–984.

[4,5]DiBaise, J, et al. Gut microbiota and its possible relationship with obesity. Mayo Clinic Proceedings. Vol. 83, Issue 4, Pages 460-469, April 2008.

[6]Velasquez-Manoff, Moises. Are Happy Gut Bacteria Key to Weight Loss? http://www.motherjones.com/environment/2013/04/gut-microbiome-bacteria-weight-loss

Made in the USA
Charleston, SC
03 April 2014